Holistic Health:

Deep Breathing To Help Relieve Chronic Pain

An All-Natural Method For Better Pain Management

RON KNESS

Contents

Disclaimer

This publication is for informational purposes only and is not intended as medical advice. Medical advice should always be obtained from a qualified medical professional for any health conditions or symptoms associated with them.

Every possible effort has been made in preparing and researching this material. We make no warranties with respect to the accuracy, applicability of its contents or any omissions.

Introduction

We breathe every day, this is obvious, but typically, most people breathe shallow, while deep breathing holds many healing abilities for the body and mind.

One significant benefit of deep breathing is pain management. A great example is the carefully crafted breath work used to manage labor pain.

A woman in labor breathes deep and short for several reasons, but a big part of that heavy breathing helps ease the pain of giving birth. The deep breathing also helps the mother see through the pain, alleviate the anxiety and stress caused by the intense pain to 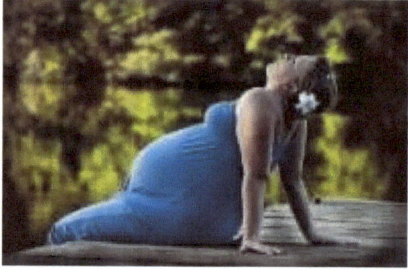 calm her mind and body so she can bring a baby into the world.

Deep breathing is a natural holistic method of pain management, and learning to deep breathe can help you manage chronic pain no matter how severe, and will therefore help to improve your quality of life. Let's get started!

What is Chronic Pain?

C hronic pain is pain that lasts longer than six months and can't be cured, but can be treated and managed. The pain can range from mild to excruciating and can be either episodic or continuous.

According to WebMD, approximately 100 million Americans alone suffer from chronic pain; imagine the numbers worldwide!

Chronic Pain Can Happen At Any Age

Chronic pain can affect anyone at any age, for example, if you have a sports injury at a young age, the pain can sometimes follow you throughout life or you are 60 and diagnosed with arthritis … the stage I'm now at in my life having been diagnosed with osteoarthritis five years ago.

Often early injuries, present injuries, or other reasons end up causing chronic pain. Some people have certain genetic codes predispose them towards having chronic pain.

There are several conditions that cause chronic pain such as fibromyalgia, arthritis, neuropathy, carpal tunnel syndrome, migraines, and others.

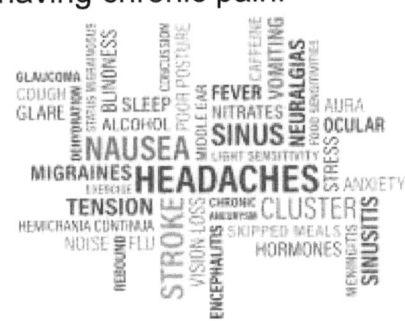

You can also have an injury when you are younger and have chronic pain stemming from it but starting later on in life.

Chronic pain can be a result of repetition in body movement from a job and sometimes, people simply suffer from chronic pain syndrome whose cause cannot be identified. Regardless, it can have a mind of its own, flaring up for no apparent reason with science still not fully understanding why.

So the best treatment is to try and manage it. While many try medications, sometimes their side effects are worse that the pain they are trying to manage. Others go for a more holistic method of treatment. It is cheaper, can be done anytime, doesn't have harmful side effects, and in some cases can be just as effective.

The Impact of Chronic Pain on Quality of Life

Your quality of life is negatively affected when you have to live with chronic pain. Going out becomes a problem, work can suffer, simple trips to the grocery store can prove difficult and enjoying time with family or even playing with kids can be a hardship.

Many find it difficult to do the things they used to do, or even to perform in their everyday lives. Unfortunately, the effects of living with pain are not limited to the physical.

Depression Associated with Chronic Pain

Depression is common in those who deal with chronic pain. The pain itself can cause a depressive state, as well as the diminished quality of life and the inability to "do" can cause depression to set in over time. It can be depressing when you want enjoy yourself and pain interferes.

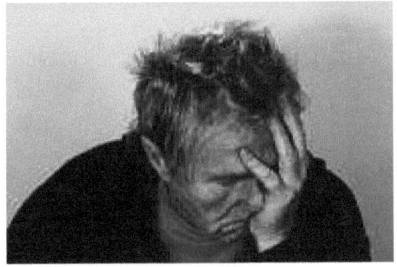

It is important to get immediate help for chronic pain. You and your doctor or holistic practitioner can devise a plan to help you live with the chronic pain and make it manageable. There are many methods of treatment, and many natural methods that can help as well.

Conventional medicine offers treatment options for pain, but some are better than others as is the case with prescription painkillers. But they have their drawbacks too.

The Problem With Prescription Painkillers

Prescription medication, such as opiates are often prescribed for pain conditions, in fact, painkillers are the most prescribed medications in the United States. They are also the most abused and cause serious and widespread addiction problems.

Painkillers temporarily hide chronic pain, but do not really "cure" it on a long-term basis. Sometimes prescription medications can cause more harm than good to a patient's overall health. Long term use causes tolerance and their effectiveness after a while wears off, thus requiring the need for higher doses to reach the same level of effectiveness. Eventually, this can lead to a physical addiction to these medications that is very difficult to overcome.

Painkillers also have uncomfortable side effects, such as drowsiness and fatigue that interfere with everyday performance. Ask your doctor a lot of questions before starting their use.

However, there are natural ways to cope with pain, including deep breathing, that can offer an alternative and all natural method to manage your pain.

A Natural Remedy Plan for Pain

Doctors and especially holistic practitioners have found that a well-rounded approach is the most effective method in managing chronic pain.

This includes using natural remedies such as garlic and turmeric as anti-inflammatories along with mind-body practices like yoga and meditation and strength building exercises. Warm baths, massage, acupuncture, and taking 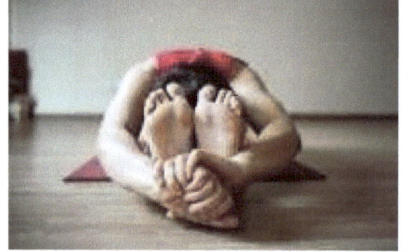 frequent rests throughout the day can help to effectively manage pain.

It is found that eating a diet of mostly vegetables, lean proteins, whole grains, nuts and fruits, and eliminating or reducing sugar intake helps to keep inflammation down to keep pain to a minimum, and supports a stronger body and immune system.

Natural remedies also involve practices such as deep breathing, which is a very simple and easy habit to get into and one that can be easily incorporated into a well-rounded pain management plan.

What is Deep Breathing?

Many people shallow breathe. Shallow breathing is simply breathing from the chest. Shallow breathing is enough to keep anyone alive and functioning, but the body can work much more efficiently with deep breathing.

Deep breathing involves breathing from the diaphragm and the abdomen with longer, stronger, and deeper breaths. Here is one example:

How To Deep Breathe

- Let go of all thoughts

- Slowly breathe in through your nose for about 4 seconds

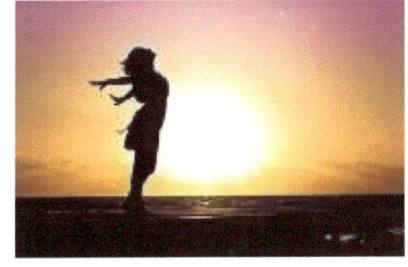

- Hold that breath for about 7 seconds

- Exhale through the mouth at twice the speed it took to inhale for 8 seconds

This practice should be repeated several times per day and also as needed when pain arises or worsens.

Benefits of Deep Breathing

Deep breathing is an excellent practice that promotes better health and provides various benefits including helping you to manage chronic pain regardless of its source. Here are nine benefits derived from deep breathing:

1. **Supports cell regeneration** – Chronic pain can inhibit the creation of new cells.

2. **Helps to clear and calm the mind** – Calmness plays a key role in pain perception.

3. **Removes toxins from the body** – This occurs as a natural result of the up and down movement of the diaphragm during deep breathing.

4. **Carbon dioxide is removed through breathing -** When you deep breathe you are getting clean oxygen to the depths of your lungs.

5. **Circulation is improved when you deep breathe** – Pumping oxygen-rich blood through your body as a result of deep breaths helps improve blood circulation.

6. **Deep breathing improves mood** – Deep breathing reduces feelings of tension, anger, and depression. You can use these deep breathing exercises to stop and regain your thoughts and alleviate negative emotions, which can exasperate pain.

7. **Releases the body's natural endorphins** – These natural painkillers help to alleviate and reduce pain.

8. **Deep breathing reduce perception of chronic pain**
   - One study, (Busch V, et al) found deep and slow breathing in concert with relaxation to be "an essential feature in the modulation of sympathetic arousal and pain perception." Studies and people who practice deep breathing report that both deep breathing exercises and meditation involving a mindful focus and a deep concentration on the breath doesn't necessarily take the pain away, but changes the perception of it so it becomes more tolerable. A lot of the fear and stress related to pain is lost through deep breathing, so while it may persist, it actually seems much less acute.

9. **Reduces stress, which consequently reduces pain**
   - Deep breathing relaxes the body, and slows the nervous system, a response opposite to what is caused by stress (fight or flight). By inducing the relaxation response and stimulating 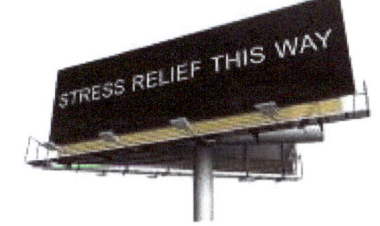 the parasympathetic nervous system, deep breathing relaxes the entire body, reduces stress reactions, and therefore reduces the perception of pain.

There really is no reason not to deep breathe on a regular basis.

It is absolutely free. It has no side effects and no dangers, but only major benefits, which reach beyond that of pain management.

For those suffering from chronic pain, deep breathing can really help, and will not only distract you from the pain, but when integrated into an overall holistic wellness plan can greatly improve pain management efforts and improve your quality of life.

How to Deep Breathe

Deep breathing exercises can be done by anyone at any fitness level. It doesn't require any special equipment and you can do it just about anywhere when you feel the need arise.

Deep breathing involves breathing through your abdomen rather than simple chest breathing. When you breathe through your abdomen, you can get a deeper breath that goes further into your lung tissue, allowing greater oxygenation.

The exercises generally involve taking a deep breath through your nose, holding it for a few seconds, and then breathing out through your mouth. A single deep breathing cycle lasts about 19 seconds—four seconds for inhalation, a 7-second hold, and 8 seconds for exhalation.

Tips To Improve Deep Breathing

Start with a deep inhalation through your nose. Use your diaphragm to expand your abdomen and to fill your lungs with oxygen. This should just take about four seconds.

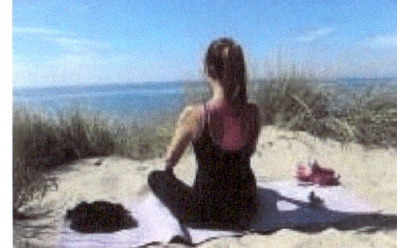

Hold the breath and count for seven seconds. Allow yourself to feel the energy build up inside you.

Then exhale fully though your mouth. This exhalation should be done over a period of about eight seconds.

Focus on relaxing your muscles and feeling the oxygen flowing throughout your body.

Repeat for another breath and do this for at least 5-10 minutes for the maximum benefit.

Make sure to set aside a minimum of two 10-minute periods of time in your day just for deep breathing exercises. Make deep breathing a priority.

Do deep breathing exercises in the morning to bring you extra energy and do it again later in the day, when you are trying to wind down and need a few minutes of relaxation.

Repeat as needed throughout the day, especially during times of stress, for pain flare-ups or simply to rejuvenate.

Deep Breathing Exercises for Pain

There are a few different breathing exercises for chronic pain besides the 4:7:8 method, but the first thing you want to do is be aware of your natural way you breathe.

Place your hand on your abdomen and breathe naturally. If nothing is happening with your abdomen, then place your hand on your chest. If your chest is moving up and down then you are shallow breathing.

Deep breathing is breathing from your diaphragm. This is what makes your abdomen go up and down. Get in the habit of diaphragm breathing by practicing every day.

Deep Breathing Exercise #1

- Lie down on the floor and point your toes up toward the sky.

- Press your shoulders down and your heels down and at the same time press your back, butt, and thighs in to the floor.

- Breathe in through your nose, hold for ½ a second, and then breathe out through your mouth. Repeat at least ten times.

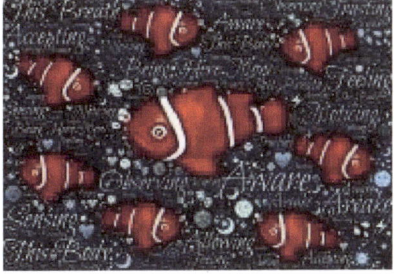

You can repeat this exercise at least three times a day and it will help alleviate stress help get toxins out of your body. If you have a hard time lowering yourself to the ground, then ask for help or use stable furniture as a prop. It is important that you lie on a hard surface.

You can also do these exercises on a couch or the bed, but they are much more effective if you lie on the carpet or yoga mat. The hard surface is part that helps you breathe better.

Deep Breathing Exercises #2

This exercise requires a chair that supports your whole body, including a wide seat, a tall back that supports your head and a design that allows your feet to be firmly planted on the ground. Any large office chair will do, but you can also buy a high back dining armchair as well. You can call it your breathing chair.

Exercise Steps

- Sit in such a chair with your arms resting on both sides and a tall back that can support your head.

- Scoot your butt to the back of the chair and make sure your head and arms are supported.

- Look straight ahead of you and keep your feet flat on the ground.

- Press your whole body into the chair and press your feet into the ground.

- Relax at the same time. Make sure your arms are well supported on the armrests.

- Close your eyes and inhale slowly through your nose to the count of about 4 seconds, making sure you're breathing in from your diaphragm and abdomen and at the same time raise your hands above your head.

- Hold your breath to the count of two and exhale though your mouth to the count of ten and at the same time bring your arms back down to the armrest.

Deep Breathing Exercises #3

Wherever you are, wherever you go you can take this exercise with you and keep doing it as much as you like, with some breaks in between. This breathing exercise is for when you are either very stressed or start feeling pain.

Exercise Steps

- When possible choose a place that has the freshest air possible.

- Breathe in through your nose and imagine a picture that means life to you whether it be an ocean, a tree, or your child - it does not matter just picture it as you are inhaling deeply through your nose; hold the fresh air for a second.

- Exhale through your mouth and as you exhale through your mouth, imagine the tiny particles releasing back into the air.

- As you exhale, the particles represent the pain, the toxins, and any negativity being released out of you.

You can repeat this exercise as many times you wish.

Making Deep Breathing A Habit

Deep breathe up to six times a day breaking it up from the early morning until the end of the day. The exercises mentioned above can be incorporated into your six daily deep breathing moments. You can choose which ones you want to do.

You can also do the simple 4:7:8 deep breathing routine anytime and anywhere throughout the day, and especially during times of stress and increased pain.

Learn them all and rotate them; soon deep breathing can become a reflex for you that will go in rhythm with your daily routine.

Having deep breathing a part of your daily routine to better live with chronic pain is one of the best ways to fight chronic pain from overtaking your life. Let deep breathing help you get your life back. Now let's look at 50 more ways deep breathing benefits your health besides reducing chronic pain.

50 Ways Deep Breathing Benefits Your Health

Here are 50 ways deep breathing and deep breathing exercises benefit your health, for optimal wellness in mind and body.

1. **Deep breathing helps detoxify the body and helps to release pent up toxins.** According to some research studies, deep breathing can release as many as 70 percent of the toxins in your body. Deep breathing exercises are effective in ridding your body of toxins that can negatively affect your health.

2. **It releases carbon dioxide.** Carbon dioxide is a normal part of cellular metabolism. When you practice deep breathing, it allows your lungs to fully exhale the buildup of carbon dioxide in your bloodstream. 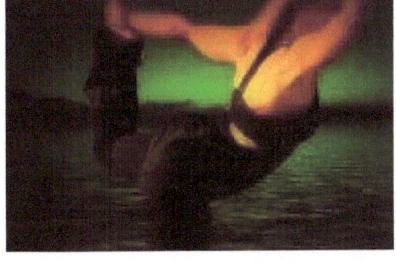 Excesses of carbon dioxide can negatively affect your health, resulting in conditions such as metabolic acidosis, which basically means that you have too much carbon dioxide in your system.

3. **Reduces tension in the body.** When you practice deep breathing, it helps loosen tight muscles and releases the tension that can build up from excess stresses in your life. This means less aches and pains!

4. **Fights the "fight or flight response."** When you are under excess stress, your adrenal glands give off norepinephrine, epinephrine, and cortisol—all hormones that increase your blood sugar, blood pressure, and respiratory rate, among other things. This is known as the "fight or flight response." Deep breathing counteracts this function of the sympathetic nervous system so you have decreased levels of these hormones and will consequently reduce your risks for the many health ramifications of chronic stress.

5. **Oxygenates your system.** Everyone needs oxygen in order for proper cellular metabolism and maximal ability of the organs in the system to do their job. Deep breathing bathes each cell and each organ in oxygen so that you can function at your maximal capacity.

6. **Brings clarity to your mind.** When you are under excessive anxiety, your brain does not get the oxygen it needs to think properly and have maximum clarity. When you pay attention to your breathing and practice deep breathing exercises, you fully 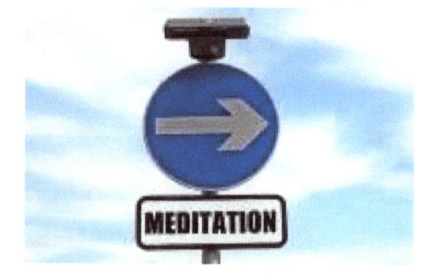 oxygenate your brain, which enhances your ability to think and allows the brain to have optimal clarity.

7. **Helps to relieve your mind of emotional difficulties.** Deep breathing can clear your mind of pent up emotions that will adversely affect your life.

Deep breathing helps release endogenous endorphins, which are the major hormones that help you feel better. Exercise will also do this but deep breathing is more efficient and relies less on your physical abilities.

8. **Counteracts pain in the body.** As mentioned, deep breathing raises your levels of endogenous endorphins the body's natural painkillers.

    Endogenous endorphins not only improve wellbeing but also decrease the perception of pain. When you engage in deep 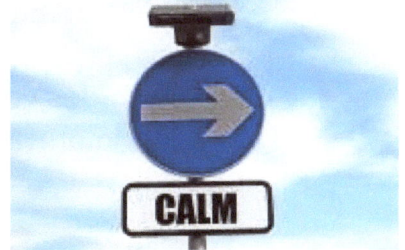 breathing, the endogenous endorphins act on pain centers of the brain so that you don't feel pain in the same way. It helps you overcome brain signals that indicate you are feeling pain so that your perception of pain is diminished.

9. **Affects abdominal organs.** When you practice deep breathing, your diaphragm moves up and down. When it does this, it massages your liver, small intestines, pancreas, and stomach. Above the level of the diaphragm, deep breathing also massages your heart. This causes an increase in circulation to these areas of your body so that they function better.

10. **Tones the abdominal muscles.** If you practice deep breathing by doing abdominal breathing (as opposed to chest breathing), you strengthen and tone the muscles of your abdomen.

    It can't promise a nice "six pack" on your abdomen

but your muscles will function better so you can do activities that require strong abdominal musculature.

11. **Improves muscle mass.** As mentioned, deep breathing affects the strength of your abdominal muscles. However, did you know it also improves the strength of your other muscles as well? Deep breathing provides oxygen to the muscles of your body and not just those involved in the breathing process. You will be stronger and will be able to exercise better. This is because the breathing exercise provides valuable oxygen to all the muscles of the body, improving their growth and maximizing their activity.

12. **Improves the immune system.** The oxygen you provide to the cells of your body also applies to the cells of the immune system. Your immune cells need as much oxygen as the rest of the cells of your body and, when they get the nutrients and oxygen provided by deep breathing, these cells work better, and your immune system is enhanced.

13. **Encourages good posture.** Depending on the way you practice deep breathing, this practice can improve your posture. You need good posture to practice deep breathing exercises so that the muscles of your chest and abdomen can effectively provide oxygen to your system. Poor posture doesn't allow you to breathe to the best of your ability; only through good posture can deep breathing truly be effective.

14. **Improves blood quality.** When you engage in deep breathing exercises, you provide oxygen to the blood cells of the body, which in turn function better. Oxygen is carried through the blood and, when you are breathing fully, oxygenation is carried to all cells of the body, including those of your blood and immune system.

15. **Maximizes your digestive process.** The more oxygen you have in your system, the better your digestive tract works. Your digestive organs (the stomach, small intestine, liver, gallbladder, and pancreas) need oxygen to perform to their maximal capacity so you absorb nutrients better. When you absorb nutrients better, it helps all of the cells of the body to function in all cellular capacities.

16. **Improves the function of your nervous system.** Your nervous system includes your brain, your spinal cord, and your peripheral nerves. When you practice deep breathing exercises, you improve the ability of your nervous system to operate at maximal capacity. These organs cannot thrive without oxygen and deep breathing is the best way to receive it.

17. **Makes your lungs stronger.** Your lungs are the major organ involved in deep breathing. When you practice deep breathing exercises, you strengthen the lungs so they exchange oxygen for carbon dioxide more efficiently. Deep breathing also opens up the alveoli of the lungs so you have fewer problems with the deeper structures of the lungs.

18. **Strengthens the heart.** Just like other cells of the body need oxygen to function, so does the heart. When the heart has plenty of oxygen through deep breathing, the cells of the heart function better, and the heart, (which is just a muscle after all) will be stronger and will function at maximal capacity.

19. **Lowers blood pressure.** Deep breathing decreases stress, which has the physiological function of lowering your blood pressure. This takes extra stress off your heart, which will not have to beat against the high pressure of the body (as happens when you have high blood pressure).

20. **Helps improve your weight in overweight people.** If you happen to be overweight and practice deep breathing exercises, your body burns fat more efficiently. This causes you to lose weight.

21. **Improves weight in underweight people.** If you happen to be underweight, deep breathing helps provide precious oxygen to those tissues of the body that are starving of nutrients and oxygens, and helps the body gain the necessary weight so 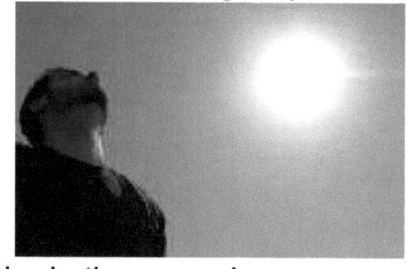 that your body weight can be in the normal range.

22. **Increase energy levels.** The practice of deep breathing energizes the body and mind so that you can have the extra energy you need to exercise or to simply go about your normal daily activities.

23. **Maximizes your stamina.** You need strong, oxygenated cells in order to have the stamina you need to partake in your daily activities. A few minutes of deep breathing per day can improve your stamina so that you can go further and longer without having to recharge your body's batteries.

24. **Improves the regeneration of your cells.** Your body is making and breaking down cells all the time. This takes cellular energy and cellular energy requires oxygen. The process of cellular regeneration needs all the oxygen it can get. Deep breathing can positively affect the cellular regeneration process by giving your system the oxygen it needs to do this job.

25. **Helps treat depression.** Depression comes from having low levels of certain neurotransmitters in the brain, particularly norepinephrine and serotonin. Deep breathing can increase the levels of oxygen in the brain so that the levels of these hormones can improve. This effectively blocks depressive symptoms.

26. **Reduces anxiety.** Anxiety often comes from an exaggerated response to stress. Deep breathing lowers stress levels so that your experience is one of calmness and peacefulness so that you experience less anxiety and can function better in daily activities.

27. **Improves self-image.** When you breathe deeply and practice deep breathing exercises, your body will change so that your abdomen is flat and you have stronger muscles that are more toned and look better.

This enhancement in your appearance can improve the way you look in the mirror and can benefit your self-image.

28. **Prevents shortness of breath.** Some cases of shortness of breath are due to shallow chest breathing, which doesn't inflate your lungs all the way. Only through deep breathing exercises can you feel that you are breathing maximally and this has the effect of making you feel less short of breath.

29. **Lowers your heart rate.** The act of deep breathing and the participation in deep breathing exercises maximizes the efficiency of the heart so that you need fewer heartbeats to do the same job as could be done if you weren't deep breathing. A slower heart rate naturally means you have a better functioning heart.

30. **It's relaxing.** When you are under too much stress, a few minutes of deep breathing exercises can relax you so your body can reset itself in a calmer way so you can go about your daily life with a better sense of relaxation.

31. **Relieves stress.** There is altogether too much stress in our daily lives. It comes from financial stressors, relationship stressors, and work stressors, just to name a few. When you practice deep breathing, your perception of stress is less and you can go about your day free of the emotional disability that comes from being under too much stress.

32. **Relaxes your muscles.** When you practice deep breathing exercises, you focus on the muscles of your abdomen and your diaphragm.

This has the natural effect of reducing the tension in the rest of your muscles so that you are more relaxed and your muscles will be less tense.

33. **Helps the fetus grow better in pregnancy.** If you are pregnant, nothing could be better than deep breathing. Deep breathing provides oxygen to the growing fetus so that it can grow and develop better under the oxygen you provide it through deep breathing. Deep breathing exercises are good things to partake in 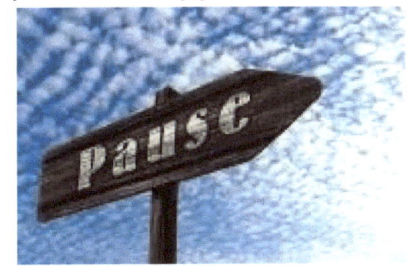 no matter what stage of pregnancy you are in.

34. **Helps reduce aching joints.** When you practice deep breathing exercises, you give your body a better sense of calm so that you relax your joints. After the deep breathing exercises are finished, your joints will be less achy and you will be able to function better in activities of daily living without arthritis symptoms.

35. **Can help a woman in labor.** If you are pregnant and practice deep breathing exercises, you can better prepare you for the intense concentration and breathing necessary to get through labor. The time to practice deep breathing exercises is when you are in your third trimester of pregnancy. This prepares you for labor so you may not need to have pain-relieving drugs during labor.

36. **Helps you with mindfulness.** Mindfulness is nothing more than staying in the present and avoiding the stressors of the past and future.

Deep breathing exercises help you stay present in time so you don't focus so much on past traumas or future worries.

37. **Can prevent miscarriages.** If you are pregnant and under too much stress, this can provoke a spontaneous miscarriage. By doing deep breathing exercises, you can better reduce the stress in the first trimester of pregnancy, which has positive effects on the pregnancy and decreases the chances that you will have a miscarriage.

38. **Reduces cortisol levels.** High cortisol levels can increase your glucose levels and promotes the deposition of fat in your fatty tissues. Deep breathing exercises will lower your cortisol levels by de-stressing you so you will have a decreased chance of suffering the negative effects of high cortisol levels.

39. **Can prevent diabetes.** Diabetes can be precipitated by stress. This is because stress can increase your cortisol levels (as mentioned above), which in turn increases your blood glucose values. There seems to be a positive correlation with stress and type 2 diabetes. The more deep breathing you do, the better able you are to have lower blood glucose levels and a decreased chance of having diabetes.

40. **Improves cognition.** When you practice deep breathing exercises, you can fully oxygenate your brain so that the nerve cells are better oxygenated. This causes you to think more clearly and reduces the stress that can cause you to have poor thought processes.

41. **Improves memory.** Your hippocampus is responsible for your short-term memory and your ability to turn short-term memories into long-term memories. When your hippocampus is better oxygenated, you remember things more clearly and you have a better chance of remembering things in your daily life.

42. **Improves sleep.** When you practice deep breathing exercises just before going to bed, you can begin to relax more into a restful state that improves your ability to fall asleep and to stay asleep during the night.

43. **Can help the lymph system.** Just as deep breathing can increase circulation; it can increase the flow of lymph fluid in the lymph system. The lymph system is responsible for finding pathogens and other harmful substances and sending these things to the lymph nodes where they can be properly processed and gotten rid of. Deep breathing can help this process along.

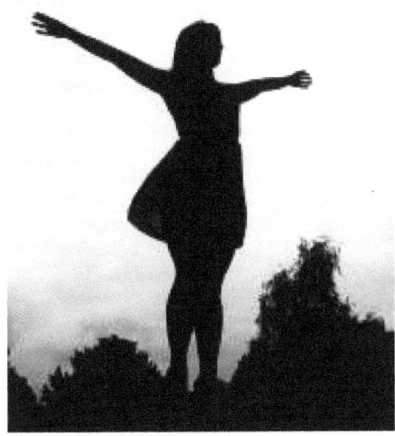

44. **Can help with asthma and chronic bronchitis.** In both of these diseases, the lungs have narrowed airways and increased lung congestion.

Deep breathing can clear out lung congestion so you are better able to cough up mucus and prevent complications of asthma and chronic bronchitis.

Patients with emphysema can also benefit from deep breathing exercises.

45. **Can improve vision.** Deep breathing can help increase the oxygen flow to the retina, which is the "seeing" part of the eye. When the retina is well oxygenated, it functions at its best and can pick up light sources that ultimately travel through the retinal system and into the brain.

46. **Can aid wound healing.** Wound healing depends on an adequate immune system and the substrates to create collagen that ultimately forms the scar that indicated a wound has healed. All of this depends on good oxygenation, which can be achieved through deep breathing exercises.

47. **Affects flexibility.** When you improve the oxygenation and blood flow to your joints and muscles, you move easier and your musculoskeletal system is less tense. This allows your joints, muscles, ligaments, and tendons to be more relaxed so your flexibility improves. This allows you to move better with a decreased risk of injury.

48. **Improves concentration.** Any time you need to concentrate on a difficult task, take a few minutes to practice deep breathing exercises. This will oxygenate your brain and decrease detracting thoughts so that you can function better with an increase in concentration.

You will be able to concentrate on the task at hand without losing your focus.

49. **Enhances your ability to learn.** If you are trying to memorize something important or are learning a new subject, the facts can be jumbled to the point where you have difficulty assimilating new information. The best way to handle this is to take a few minutes to practice deep breathing exercises so that you can learn what you need to learn.

50. **Can decrease wrinkles.** By increasing the blood flow to the skin, you can fill the skin tissue with more fluid. This smooths wrinkles so that your physical appearance can be improved. Deep breathing can allow this increase in circulation to occur so, when you look into the mirror, you have fewer wrinkles and will be more pleased with your appearance.

Meditation

According to Dr. Patricia Bloom, director of integrated health programs at the Mount Sinai Medical Center in New York, a wide array of research in neuroscience finds meditation to play a key role in effective pain management. In many cases, meditation has allowed patients to stop using prescription painkillers.

What Is Meditation

Meditation is breathing while being still. It involves a deep focus on the breathe, or an object, sometimes it uses mantras, mindfulness or guided imagery and visualization.

It has many benefits for the body and mind, and is certainly a wonderful addition to a holistic pain management plan.

There are many ways to meditate; the key is find those that work for you and practice regularly.

Final Thoughts

C hronic pain can really diminish your quality of life. For some it is severely debilitating and interferes with every day activities and just being able to perform the necessary tasks of life.

It can really be a terrible thing to live with. Sometimes, the worst part is that conventional medicine has little answers and no cure. This is one of the reasons that a holistic approach that integrates various natural methods to manage pain is one your best options in dealing with it.

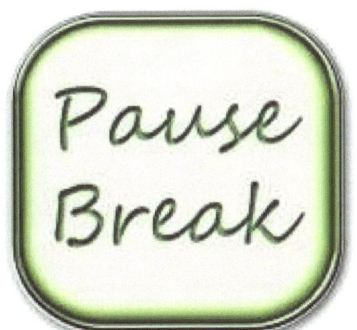

Chronic pain can make you feel helpless and frustrated, and can lead to depression. A holistic pain management plan may be the answer to improve your quality of life and feel better.

Deep breathing has been used for years in meditation and other mind-body practices, such as yoga and Tai Chi and has been found to help chronic pain.

You will need to make some effort to make it a habit and allow it to become a part of your natural routine. It may feel a little funny at first, but eventually it will become second nature and a routine part of your daily life.

Deep breathing is a great addition to a well-rounded pain management plan, it has no side effects, it's free, and it helps. Get started today!

Stay well and take care!

Other Health and Fitness Books by This Author

If you would like to read more about Senior Health and Fitness, here is a list of the <u>titles, CreateSpace links and descriptions:</u>

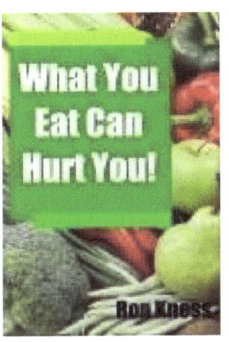

What You Eat Can Hurt You

https://www.createspace.com/4963196

Do you know that certain foods increase your risk for inflammation, disease and illness? It's true! And certain foods can help cure and heal you if you do get sick. Knowing which foods to eat and which ones to avoid empowers you to manage your own health.

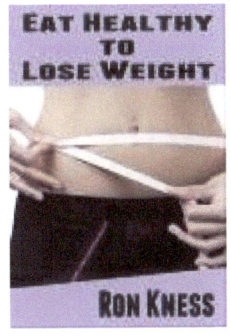

Eat Healthy to Lose Weight

https://www.createspace.com/4962939

As you read through our book, we show you which foods you should and should not be eating to reach your weight loss goal, along with discussing how to maintain your weight loss and stay within a few pounds of your goal weight. Banish the weight you keep gaining back each time by learning how to live a healthy lifestyle.

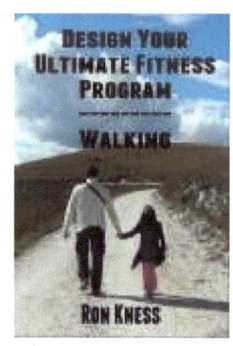

Design Your Ultimate Fitness Program - Walking

https://www.createspace.com/5252272

In my book Design Your Ultimate Fitness Program – Walking, we discuss the considerations that need to be made when designing a custom walking program, along with:

• Equipment needed
• Wearable technology you can use to track your walking
• And how to make walking more challenging

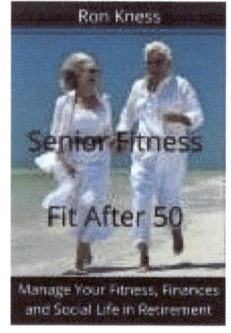

Senior Fitness – Fit After 50: Learn How to Manage Your Fitness, Finances and Social Life in Retirement

https://www.createspace.com/5474751

Inside you will discover answers to your most pressing questions:
• What do I need to know about downsizing my home?
• What are the best tips for staying healthy as you approach your 50's?
• When should I start planning for retirement?
• I am worried about being lonely once I retire, do others feel the same?
• Is it worthwhile to carry two homes during retirement?
And more…

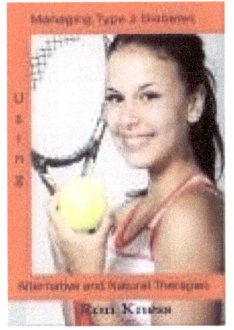

Managing Type 2 Diabetes Using Alternative And Natural Therapies

https://www.createspace.com/5401244

While Type 2 diabetes can be managed medically, there are many alternative natural and holistic methods of therapy and treatment that can further enhance quality of life and minimize the effects of this disease. In this book, I discuss 12 different types, including yoga, reflexology and acupuncture to name just three.

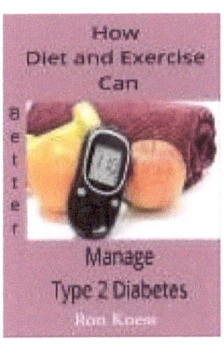

How Diet and Exercise Can Better Manage Type 2 Diabetes

https://www.createspace.com/5404845

Of the different types of diabetes, only Type 2 can be reversed. In my book How Diet and Exercise Can Better Manage Type 2 Diabetes, we reveal the three things you can do to best manage your disease, including:
• Diet
• Exercise
• Weight management

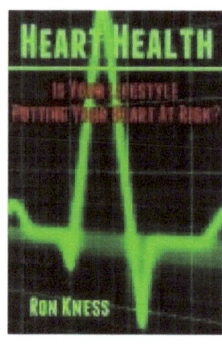

Heart Health: Is Your Lifestyle Putting Your Heart at Risk?

https://www.createspace.com/5464020

In my ebook Is Your Lifestyle Putting Your Heart At Risk? we discuss the six greatest risks to your heart and the lifestyle changes you can make to mitigate them.

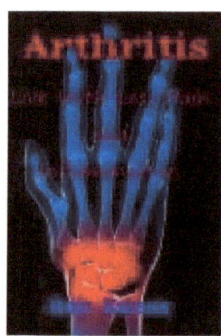

Arthritis – Live Wth Less Pain and Inflammation: Tips and Techniques You Can Use to Lessen the Pain and Inflammation

https://www.createspace.com/5457441

Discover Simple Tips & Information That Will Help Reduce The Painful Symptoms Of Arthritis!

You learn things like:
• Simple and effective information that will help you manage the pain and inflammation that comes along with arthritis, so that you can live an active, full life without debilitating pain.
• The different types of arthritis, their symptoms and how to alleviate their painful side effects.
• The pros and cons of over-the-counter arthritis medications, plus simple tips that will help you know how to choose the right supplements.
• Free, yet effective ways to get relief from arthritis pain and inflammation, so you don't have to suffer anymore.

the effects arthritis can have significant impact on your physical and mental well-being, but this books shows you how to overcome its painful symptoms and live life relatively pain free.

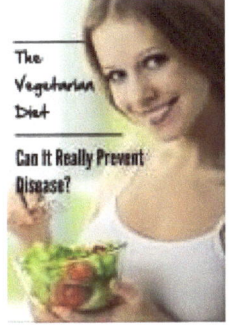

The Vegetarian Diet – Can It Really Prevent Disease?

https://www.createspace.com/5519874

Is a vegetarian diet right for you? Multiple studies have shown over and over that a vegetarian diet goes along way in preventing certain chronic diseases, such as:

• Heart Disease
• Cancer
• Diverticulitis
• Type 2 Diabetes
• Hypertension
• Obesity
• Kidney Failure

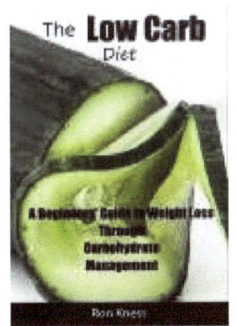

The Low Carb Diet: A Beginner's Guide to Weight Loss Through Carbohydrate Management

https://www.createspace.com/5416348

In my book "The Low-Carb Diet – A Beginners' Guide to Weight Loss Through Carbohydrate Management", I reveal a successful method of losing weight based in part on the amount and type of carbohydrates you consume.

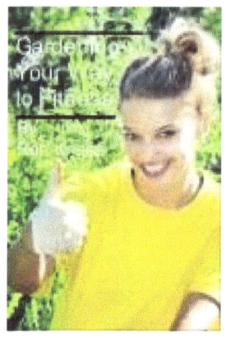

Gardening Your Way to Fitness: The Fun Way to Get Fit and Provide Beauty and Healthful Bounty for Your Family

https://www.createspace.com/5459564

The gym is a great place to stay fit during the colder seasons, but once the temperature turns warmer you want to spend more time outside. Plus, you'll have the benefit of fresh wholesome produce to enjoy by growing vegetables in your backyard garden.

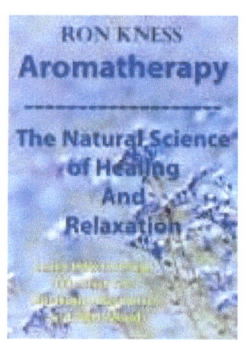

Aromatherapy - The Science of Healing and Relaxation: Learn How Essential Oils Elicit The Relaxation Response And Alter Mood

https://www.createspace.com/5714434

In my book Aromatherapy – The Science of Healing and Relaxation, we reveal the natural holistics methods you can use to heal the body from certain medical issues and to relive stress through relaxation. In particular we talk about:

• Aromatherapy - what it is and how it works

• Essential Oils – how the effects of certain aromas differs from others

• Recipes – how to make your own essential oil combinations

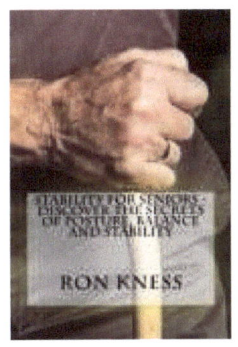

Stability for Seniors: Discover the Secrets of Posture, Balance and Stability

https://www.createspace.com/6096479

Many people sacrifice their health in pursuit of their career. They are so busy making a living that they neglect to make a life. The excuse that they do not have time to exercise is tossed about so frequently that they end up letting their health and fitness slide.

If you are not regularly active, you will have muscular atrophy over time. Your flexibility will decrease. Your core strength will diminish. As time progresses, you will be less limber and more rigid.

This is exactly how people age poorly. It's a process that has snowballed over time.

Only with regular exercise and a healthy diet can you have a body that is fit and has the ability to almost reverse aging.

If you have neglected your health for years and life seems to be a chore now because you can't get around without assistance, do not feel dejected.

You can remedy the situation. You can restore the strength, balance and stamina that you have lost. It is never too late to become what you might have been.

This guide will show you exactly what you need to do to restore your balance, strengthen your core and give you the ability to live life to its fullest. Read how …

About the Author

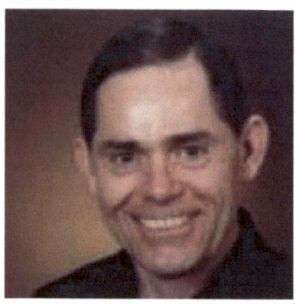 I grew up in Central Minnesota, where my parents owned and operated a fishing resort. Once out of high school I tried a couple of semesters of college, only to quit halfway through the Spring term; I decided at that time that college wasn't for me.

Then I decided to follow my father's previous occupation as an auto mechanic. I graduated from a two-year of vocational training course and worked as a mechanic. While in vocational training, I decided to join the National Guard where I eventually ended up working full-time for 32 years.

So how does all of this relate to writing? In one of my leadership schools, the instructor, who was an English teacher at a juvenile detention center, presented writing to me in a whole new way - a way that started to develop my interest in working with words.

Fast forward about 40 years and I now have over 50 books listed on Amazon for Kindle and CreateSpace.

Besides my own writing, I also ghostwrite ebooks, reports, articles, blogs and do Kindle conversions for my clients on a variety of topics.

Today my wife and I live in Gold Canyon, AZ, where you'll find me happily sitting in my office typing away on my laptop as I work on my next book or ghostwriting project . . . that is if we are not traveling on a cruise ship - our new-found mode of travel.